Shaking Hands with
CANCER

and Coming Out Fighting

by cheryl Dal Porto

photography by
Susan Ley

(The author spells her first name with a lower case c.
Read why on page 43.)

Pine Grove Publishing Company
Pine Grove, California

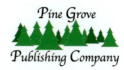
Pine Grove
Publishing Company

ISBN 978-0-9716876-1-5
by cheryl Dal Porto
Photography by Susan Ley

The information in this book is true and complete to the best of our knowledge. All recommendations are made without any guarantee on the part of the Author or Publisher, who also disclaim any liability incurred in connection with the use of this data or specific details.

The Author is not a medical practitioner; she is a cancer survivor. This book does not offer medical advice nor should any of the items discussed be substituted for instructions and advice from your medical team. The goal of this book is one of inspiration. Items discussed were and continue to be valuable to the Author and she hopes may be useful to you.

I made it a point to shake hands with the cancer,
and come out fighting.

I am not brave; I simply chose not to be scared.

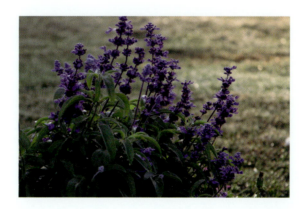

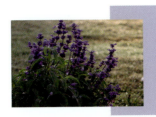

FOREWORD

It is with humility that I pen this foreword to a book written by a dear friend. My wife, Audrey, and I have shared good times and less than good times with cheryl and Bob. She is, without a doubt, a remarkable woman. She has met the challenges of life with dignity and a resolve to overcome the challenges.

She recognizes that her battle has not been, "I've won the race," rather that it is a process with a philosophy that allows her to make the best of every day. In the process, she gives light and hope to other travelers.

Although this book is about her experiences as a cancer survivor, it is more about conquering obstacles and overcoming challenges. Is there anyone who has not faced obstacles or challenges? This book is for you. The principles are the same, whether it is battling cancer, loss of a loved one, betrayal or a home destroyed by a fire.

I recall vividly the time, shortly after she received the awful news that her pap smear was positive, that she confided in me the results of the test. As a medically-trained person, I understood the gravity of her situation. I don't recall all that was said, but, in essence, I suggested she act quickly and follow the advice of her doctors. She needed a hug and I willingly obliged.

We have kept close as the years have passed by, as good friends should. Too many times I received a phone call from Bob stating that cheryl was back in the hospital for another surgery. At one point, cheryl suggested to her surgeon that he insert a zipper in her abdominal wall to make it easier to get in and out.

As important as cheryl's indomitable spirit is, it is evident that she has the support of a loving husband, her children, her mother, other family and friends, and an incredible medical team that has been there for her since the beginning.

The images that accompany this book, bring serenity and loveliness that may give solace to the troubled. May everyone with challenges to face find this book uplifting so that they, too, may come out fighting.

~Murray E. Fowler

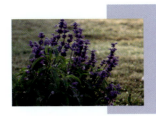

INTRODUCTION

The date was Tuesday, May 15, 1990. A beautiful spring day, and I had decided to leave the office a bit early to run by the doctor's for a scheduled gynecological examination before catching lunch and returning to an office buzzing with pending deadlines.

I never returned to my place of business that day, nor did I enjoy a quick lunch. Instead, I drove directly home ... 35 miles ... and I don't remember ever getting behind the wheel of the car!

I had been given an examination that had resulted in a diagnosis of cancer. Later it would be further explained as poorly differentiated adenosquamous carcinoma of the cervix and well differentiated papillary mesothelioma of the pelvic peritoneum.

A diagnosis of cancer can certainly ruin the most beautiful of spring days. However, I quickly learned that it's all how you respond to the devastating news that puts it back into perspective.

I was fortunate. Along with my best friend, Susan, three of my adult children were able to keep our publishing business going and with the nurturing support of my husband, Bob, and family and friends, I truly found my will - my determination - to live.

Susan and I wrote and photographed this book out of a wish and a desire to give you an alternative to the many academic books on the market. These books make necessary reading because it is knowledge and understanding that are the keys to letting go of unreasonable fears.

Therefore, read every specialized book you can get your hands on. Fill your brain with what they have to say. But leave room for SHAKING HANDS WITH CANCER - AND COMING OUT FIGHTING, and fill your heart with its offerings.

DEDICATIONS

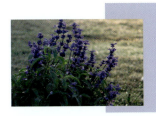

After my initial surgery for cervical cancer, I woke up the following day in the intensive care unit. I remember seeing eight sets of eyes circling the bed. They didn't speak a word, but their faces said volumes. I would soon learn that my surgeon had discovered a second cancer, and my odds of survival were not good.

During the time I had been unconscious, I clearly recall a voice whispering softly in my ear - "c'mon cheryl, come back to us, you can do it." Upon opening my eyes, I was introduced to that voice and learned that his name was Jack. He was an ICU nurse and he was not going to hear a word of defeat. He told me that I would be getting out of bed the following day, and I would be walking ... small steps at first ... but giant leaps by nightfall. The next morning, my son, Marc, was there to help lift me out of bed and to assist me in taking those first baby steps ... those crucial steps that would lead to recovery.

And so, to those eight sets of eyes - my devoted husband, Bob, my children - Cleave, Marc, Cathy and Bobby - to two of my best friends in the world - Murray and Susan - and finally, to Jack, whoever and wherever you are - I dedicate this book to you. And to my Mother who offered her support throughout the writing and publishing of this book - I also dedicate this work to you. This dedication would not be complete without thanking Susan, this book's photographer and my dear friend, for encouraging me to get my story told. And finally, and most importantly, to Bob, for being at my side every step of the way. In this journey, he has carried the majority of the load.

I love all of you.

~ cheryl

To cheryl from Susan

cheryl's gifts surround me like a string of pearls.
Each one a talisman for the years ahead.
Understanding, laughter, love and hope ...
they are all there.
Rare gifts from cheryl's world to mine.

Upon discovering a second cancer in my body, my oncologist/surgeon

of his mouth, but I heard words coming from a different voice even louder ...

I HAD TO FACE DEATH BEFORE I COULD FULLY APPRECIATE LIFE.

told my husband and I that I had very little chance of living past 3 years. I heard the words that came out

prove him wrong ... prove him wrong ... prove him wrong. That date was June 12, 1990.

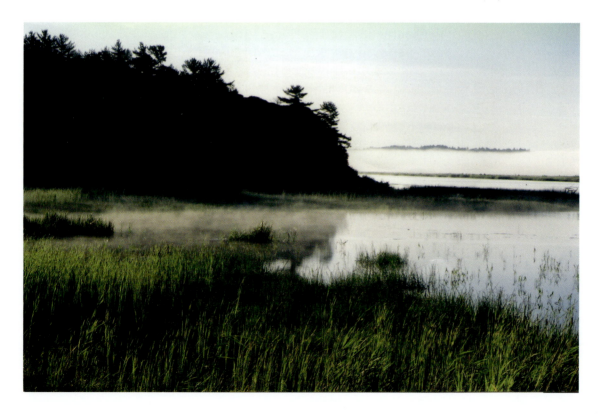

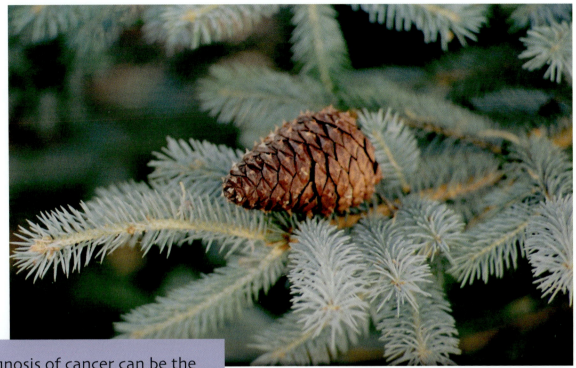

A diagnosis of cancer can be the most significant day in your life. However, it's how you respond to the devastating news that puts it back into perspective.

Since my radiation therapy was going to extend over 13 weeks, I made a calendar in order to cross off each week to see my progress. But my Mom did even better. She purchased 13 little gifts that I could choose from and open on each Friday. It was so much fun looking forward to those little boxes. And then my husband joined ranks, and began taking me out-of-town each weekend and our out-of-town excursions kept getting better and better as I advanced towards my goal. I sometimes spent the entire weekend in an inn's bathroom vomiting, but the get-aways were definitely something to look forward to.

Although cancer is usually thought of as a single disease, it is in fact more than 200 completely sepa-

But as different as the prognosis and the treatments, the facts are the same .... your need for one

CANCER IS A MENACING WORD ... SAY IT RAPIDLY ONE HUNDRED TIMES ... IT BECOMES LESS MENACING THE MORE YOU ALLOW YOURSELF TO SPEAK THE WORD.

rate diseases. However, whether it is 1st stage skin cancer or 4th stage pancreatic cancer, the word brings us to our knees.

big, significant helping of positive attitude, with sides of hope, optimism, dreams, faith, conviction and confidence.

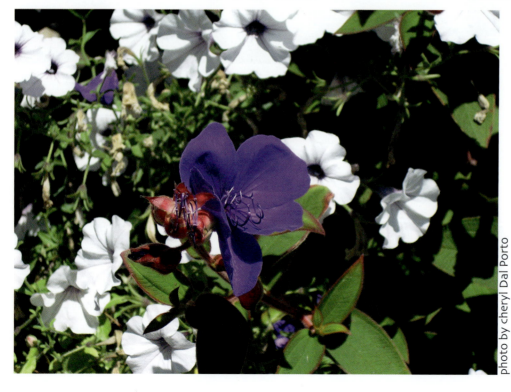

photo by cheryl Dal Porto

Shaking Hands with Cancer

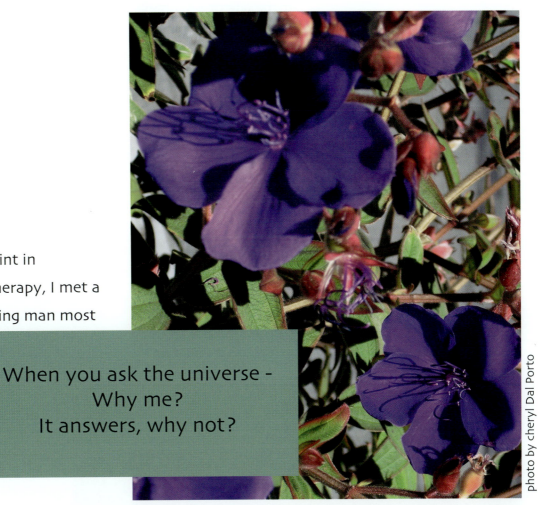
photo by cheryl Dal Porto

During my stint in radiation therapy, I met a young, good looking man most likely in his late 20's. He was tall and thin, and a picture of health.

When you ask the universe -
Why me?
It answers, why not?

In talking with him, he couldn't get past the "why me's?" He had been diagnosed with lung cancer, and he had never smoked a cigarette in his life. His chosen career had landed him in an office full of smokers, and yet it was he who had the cancer.

He eventually quit therapy and decided not to fight his disease. To this day, I remain saddened by his choice.

At the age of 43, I had my life planned. I had helped to raise four wonderful children who were now all young adults, was

And then along came cancer.

Now I look back on my well planned life and appreciate the curve ball that

SOMETIMES LIFE HAS DIFFERENT PLANS FOR US.

running my own successful publishing company, had all of the farm animals that I could possibly care for, and my husband and I were happily entering a time in our lives where we were appreciating the fruits of our labor.

it threw me. I am a better person today because of it and although I will never again believe in a well planned life, I do believe in making the most of every unplanned , beautiful day that I am alive.

About three days following one of my surgeries, my oncologist suggested that I get out of bed and walk around the ward to get as much exercise as possible. I decided to give his advice a try. I began to walk .... up and down hallways, into the

I have my doubts about predestination. However, I am a firm believer in determination.

cafeteria, by nurses' stations ... and finally, into this dark, quiet room that said, "No talking." There were probably 12 beds in all ... and every one of them was occupied by a patient who was not speaking. All you could hear was the sound of their breathing machines. It was not until I crept by one particular bed with an older man in it, that I realized where I was. It was the death room ... these people were all on their last breath. The man finally spoke to me. His words were soft, but firm. He said, "Turn around and get out of here. Fight with everything you have." Then he smiled at me, a very faint smile, and never uttered another word. By the time I was released from the hospital, he had most likely died ... but his words are forever etched in my brain. "Fight, fight, fight."

Before anyone begins chemotherapy, they are given a list of supplies to have on hand. The list will most likely include a wig garments, bath bubbles, luxurious bed sheets and pillow cases, wonderful bath toys, chocolates, uplifting quotation books,

CANCER HAS GIVEN ME FAR MORE THAN IT HAS TAKEN.

and medication for nausea. I would suggest an additional list of supplies: colorful clothing, comfortable pajamas, sexy undergarments, favorite movies, fragrant candles, journals, coloring books and the cheeriest bucket for vomiting that you can find!

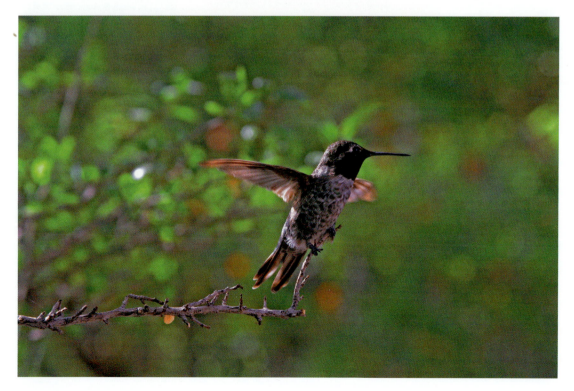

I created four small boxes that would house a variety of items. The first box was for all of the encouraging cards, letters and little mementoes that I received from friends and family. Many times, when I was especially down or weak, I would open the box and re-read all of the cheery words. The second box was labeled "letting go". On bits of paper, I would write down those things that I did not have control over, and add them to the box. I had to open this particular box on many an occasion, to remind myself that something was out of my control and that I had to give it to a higher

I knew what cancer could do to me, but not for me.

power. The third box was the primary reason I created this book. On scraps of paper I would write encouraging words to myself. When I encountered a special person during my treatments for cancer, I would add their name to the box and why I found them to be special. Finally, the fourth box. To this day …. it remains empty. This is a box I created for my husband and my children for memories they could share following my death. Tidbits for my "Celebration of Life" gathering, and perhaps things they remembered from the day of my passing. I have vowed to keep it empty for as long as possible.

My family decided that they should do everything for me while I was in treatment. They took

At first, their helpfulness came as a relief, because I was not as physically strong as I had been.

CANCER HELPED ME BECOME A FIGHTER. IT WAS A CHOICE.

turns preparing the meals, driving me to my appointments, doing farm chores and keeping up with the laundry on a daily basis.

After a few weeks, however, I began taking back my jobs, little by little, and it is at this time that I truly began to heal.

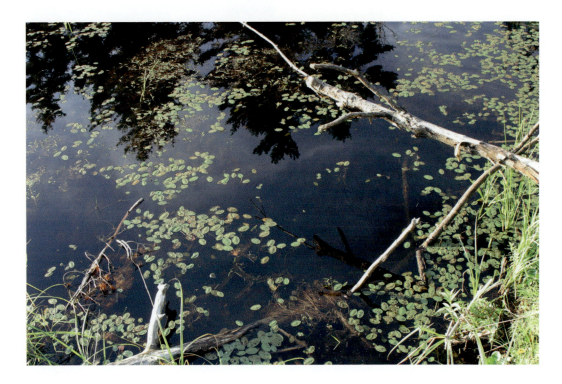

Shaking Hands with Cancer

Decide right now. Do you want to become an active participant in your battle, or do you want to sit on the sidelines, allowing all decisions to be made for you? You can begin fighting for your recovery by increasing the number of pleasant emotions within your body and decreasing those that are unpleasant. Pursue happiness with every fiber of your being, and reduce stress that can play against the fight for a cure.

I want to let you in on a secret ... cancer doesn't have to be scary. You can reverse roles with such a diagnosis, and scare the wits out of it.

I , personally, learn very little from sitting on the bench and I urge you to become partners with your physicians and other caretakers.

With cancer, you have
to move slowly through
different stages ... anger ...
grief ... loneliness ....

THINK OUTSIDE THE DIAGNOSIS.

However, don't allow
youself to get stuck in one
stage longer than necessary.

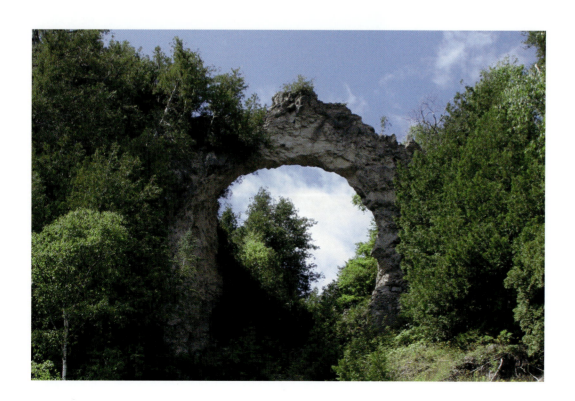

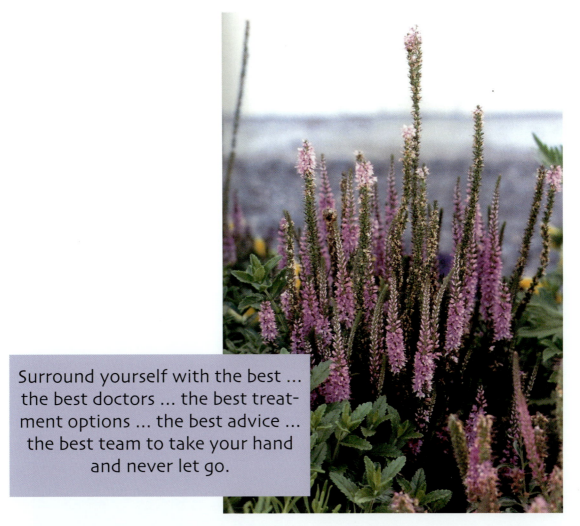

Surround yourself with the best ...
the best doctors ... the best treatment options ... the best advice ...
the best team to take your hand
and never let go.

Win over your medical team by making yourself unforgettable. Bring your own uniqueness to the situation. On a day that my doctor had to present me with bad news - and I knew it was coming - I baked cookies for him and his staff. It brought an entirely different tone to the day. My doctor, and all of his nurses, now know me on a first-name basis. In fact, when I call, they immediately know my voice. Demand that your medical team sees you as an individual, and not a statistic.

Each time my oncolo-
gist had to write me a new
prescription, he wrote one
for my husband to fill for

**CANCER WILL TAKE WHAT IT CAN.
TUG HARD ON YOUR END OF THE ROPE.**

me as well. It usually read
- "One hour of shopping at
Nordstrom" or "good for
one new pair of shoes."

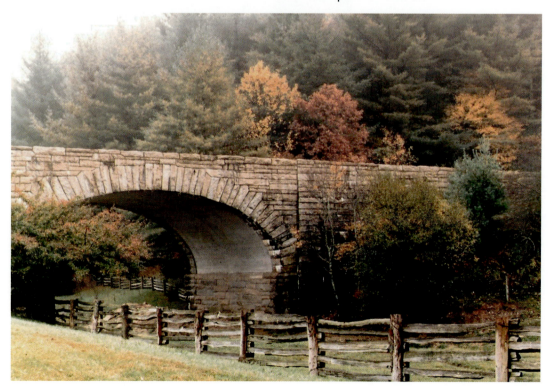

Shaking Hands with Cancer

I was subjected to 13 weeks of radiation therapy and never have I felt more like a product on an assembly line than with my daily doses of the red beam.

Before our appointments with "the machine", we were asked to change into blue hospital gowns that barely covered our back sides.

Patients filled the lobby, nervously waiting. Their eyes focused on the empty space between their two feet, numb with anticipation of the radiation.

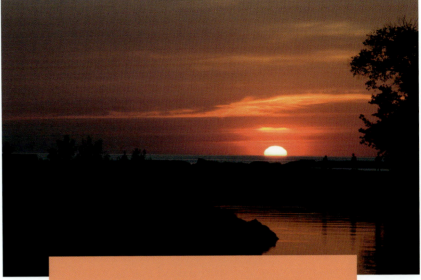

Life is more difficult with cancer. However, focus on the word life, and not on cancer.

I became determined to make this otherwise dark hour one that we might even look forward to. So, slowly, I began introducing myself to the other patients, and it wasn't long before we began opening up to each other.

By the time my 13 weeks was up, we had replaced those sterile magazines in the waiting room with tiny inspirational quotation books, we were sporting colorful neon socks with our drab blue gowns, we were drinking water out of wine goblets and we were bringing baked goodies to the staff, who could no longer feel sorry for us (we were a mighty happy group).

I actually began missing the games we had created to boost our strength ... how many words we could find in the sign Radiation Therapy (we even created a few never to be found in Webster's) and how many miles we could drive home before we vomited. The person who could drive the furthest received the loudest round of applause the following day.

One particularly hard day during radiation therapy, I asked to see my radiologist who normally only saw me at the end of each week. Once he put his hand on my shoulder and asked me to come into his office, I started sobbing like a baby.

He took out a book of poetry by e.e. cummings (I had mentioned that he was my favorite poet the week before), and began to read. After about 15 minutes, I felt strong again, and left his office. Like I said, surround yourself with the best.

AVOID CLIMBING, AND YOU WILL NEVER FALL.
BE PREPARED, HOWEVER, TO NEVER EXPERIENCE
THE SATISFACTION OF GETTING UP.

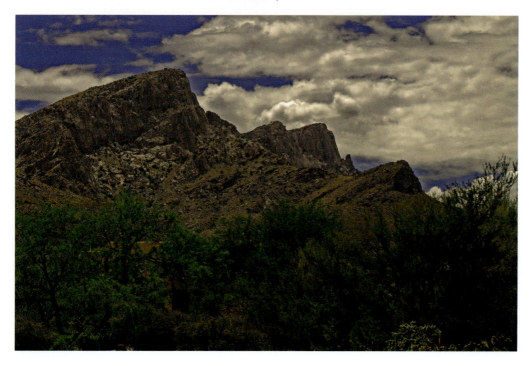

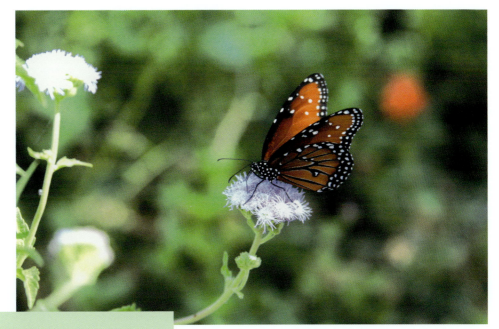

You have a big hand in writing your own life story.

In radiation therapy, I met a young woman with advanced stage lung cancer. Her prognosis was encouraging, but her doctor had told her that she had to quit smoking immediately if she was going to have a fighting chance. One day, I watched her smuggle a cigarette out of her purse and light it. She puffed away. Then she joined us in the waiting room, reeking with cigarette odor. I waited until I saw her repeat this behavior, kept watch until our eyes met and she knew that I had seen. She quickly joined me in the waiting room, and said, "Please don't tell the doctor that I am smoking. He will kill me." Who was she kidding?

Fighting cancer - any type of cancer - must be a joint effort between you and your medical team, and this partnership must be based on honesty.

Cancer starts with one abnormal cell. That cell becomes two abnormal cells that become four

start with one fear, that fear becomes two fears, that become four fears and so on. Stop the fear

STATISTICS CAN BE PROVEN WRONG.

abnormal cells and eight ... and sixteen ... and so on. As a cancer patient, you

and then you can concentrate on stopping the spread of the cancer.

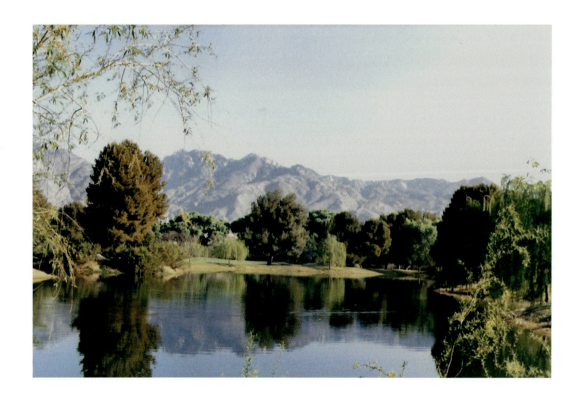

Shaking Hands with Cancer

Following my 13 weeks of radiation, and a period of time to allow my immune system to recover, I was hospitalized once again. This round of hospitalization included one week of isolation with a radiation device inserted into my cervix, and a different form of chemotherapy injected into each arm.

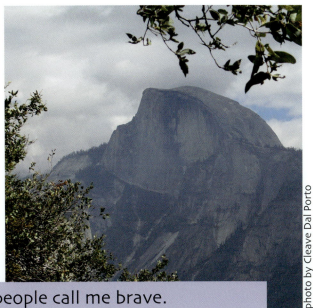

photo by Cleave Dal Porto

After I was completely hooked up, another lifeline with self-administered morphine claimed my last available vein. I was told that no one could enter the room during the next ten days, and that the nurses would check on me through a small window in the door. My husband chose not to honor the

Some people call me brave.
However, I didn't know if I had the courage to face such unimaginable pain ... day after day ... but you learn that you do what you have to do, and, hopefully, you come out on the other side a better, stronger person.

"do not enter room" sign and, therefore, exposed himself to an abnormal amount of radiation. But the staff recognized the threat, and kept outside the door, except for one nurse. After my fifth day with little human contact, she ventured into the room and gave me a big hug. I have never been so sick in all my life, and I remember asking her why she had crossed the boundary. She simply said, "You looked like you needed a hug!"

I don't remember being able to look at her nametag or even get a thank you out of my parched mouth, but I have never forgotten her. I hope that, somehow, she knows what she did for me that day.

All of us have preconceived notions about cancer. Whether it's an aunt that died from breast can- must put everything that we have collected in our minds and hearts about those cases aside.

THROW AWAY ALL PRECONCEIVED NOTIONS. FILL YOUR BRAIN WITH WHAT IS, NOT WITH WHAT ISN'T.

cer when we were in grade school or a distant cousin passing after a lengthy battle with kidney cancer, once we are diagnosed, we We must listen to our medical team and realize that our case is different from any other case of cancer.

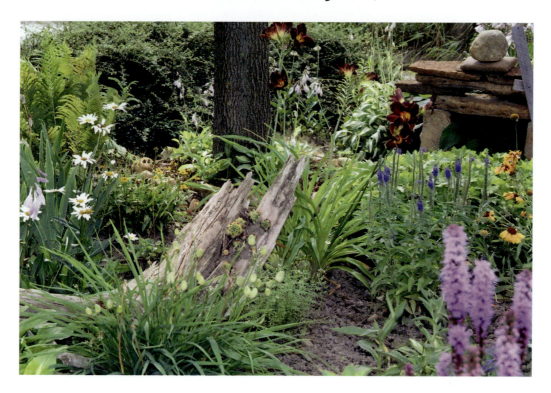

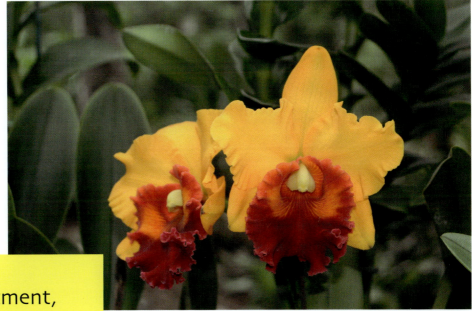

During treatment,
discover your abilities,
not your limitations.

Picture this: You are seated at a table playing cards. However, this game is a bit different from others that you have played. This particular dealer is handing out life struggles. So, the dealer deals. The first player is given a hand of child abduction. The second player is given a hand of heart attack (no warning ... no chance to fight back ... the attack is fatal). The third player is dealt rape (a family member is raped and left for dead ... she recovers physically, but never emotionally). The fourth player gets multiple sclerosis (and one day soon will be wheelchair bound). You are given the hand of cancer. Now, do you want to throw the cards back or are you going to play the hand you were dealt? I, for one, am playing...

Life is like a rainbow.
Don't lose sight of all the
hues. Cancer is just a dark-

LIFE COMES WITH AN ABSOLUTE DEATH SENTENCE.
CANCER MAY COME WITH A DEATH SENTENCE.
SEEMS LESS SCARY NOW, DOESN'T IT?

er shade co-mingling with
all of the other beautiful,
bright colors.

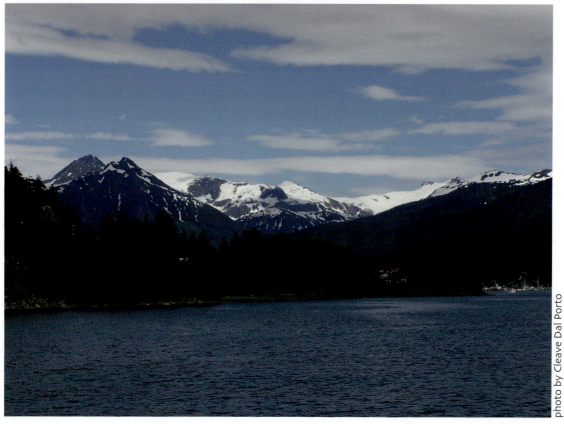

photo by Cleave Dal Porto

Shaking Hands with Cancer

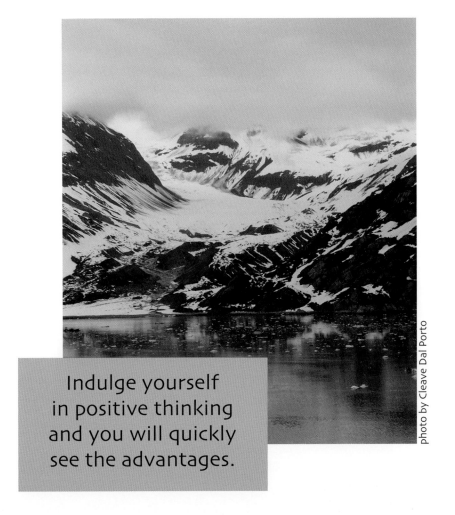

photo by Cleave Dal Porto

Indulge yourself
in positive thinking
and you will quickly
see the advantages.

Two years ago, for my 60th birthday, my husband and eleven members of our family embarked on an Alaskan cruise. We were telling my oncology nurse practitioner that we were concerned about the cruise, because if I became sick, the ship's doctor would not be familiar with my cancers and my numerous medications. She thought for a moment, and then said that she had always wanted to see Alaska. She booked herself on the same cruise.

Each time I have a birthday, I celebrate my new age. I do not wish that I was younger or more youthful looking.

DON'T EVER LET CANCER DEFINE YOU.

I celebrate each birthday knowing how many people have not had the opportunity to reach the age that I am now enjoying.

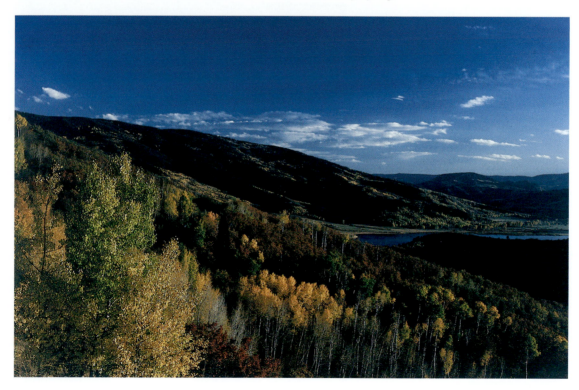

My preschool grandson accompanied me to nearly all of my post-treatment doctor appointments. "Cancer talk" was something that became second nature to him. One day after he had started school, I picked him up at the designated time. I was particularly tired that day, and I told him so. I will never forget his response. "The cancer is just acting up today, Grandma. I feel a little bit of cancer, too, so I will take a nap with you." Oh, out of the mouths of babes ....

Cancer became the starring role
in my life;
I had to learn to force it backstage.

The well-wisher knows that they want you to be healthy again and many it belongs, and where it will do the most good. Well- intentioned friends

OPTIMISM CANNOT BE TAUGHT FROM A BOOK; BUT IT CAN CERTAINLY BE DEMONSTRATED.

times, will want you to hear their advice and sug- gestions. However, put your absolute trust where and family members (and I emphasize well-inten- tioned) can drain your emotional energy.

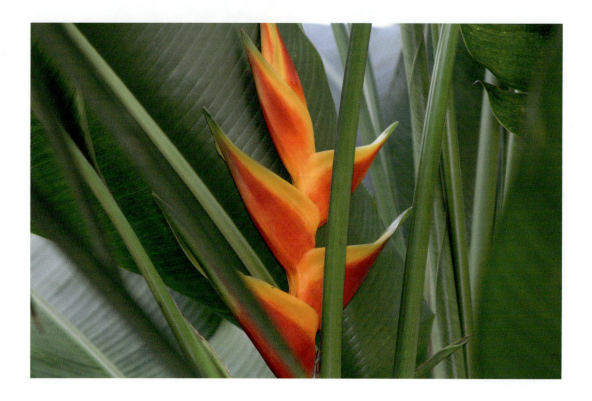

Shaking Hands with Cancer

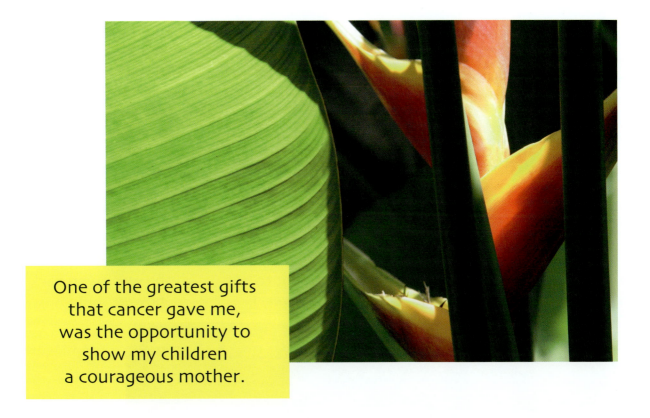

One of the greatest gifts
that cancer gave me,
was the opportunity to
show my children
a courageous mother.

I never realized it before, but most people have a difficult time looking cancer patients in the eye, and asking how they are. They wait until you are out of the room, and then whisper their concerns about your health. I was one of those people. Look cancer patients and everyone else with their own unique health issues square in the eye and say, "I am concerned about you. Please tell me how you are doing."

When I was first di-
agnosed with cancer, my
husband felt powerless.

learned that by giving my
medical team permission
to include my husband,

**DO ALL YOU CAN TO TAKE CARE OF YOURSELF
AND YOU WILL ALSO BE TAKING CARE OF YOUR PRIMARY CARETAKER.**

There was nothing that
he could do to improve
my situation, except to be
supportive. However, I

my primary caretaker,
in all decisions and news,
he was given back his
power.

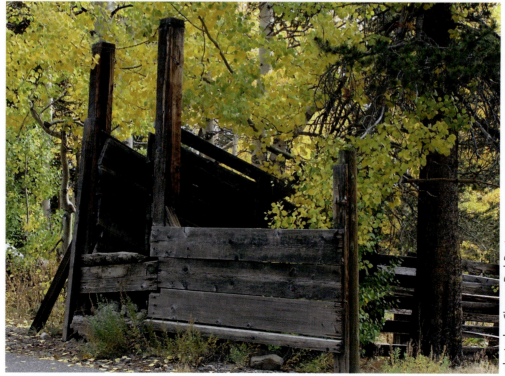

photo by Cleave Dal Porto

Shaking Hands with Cancer

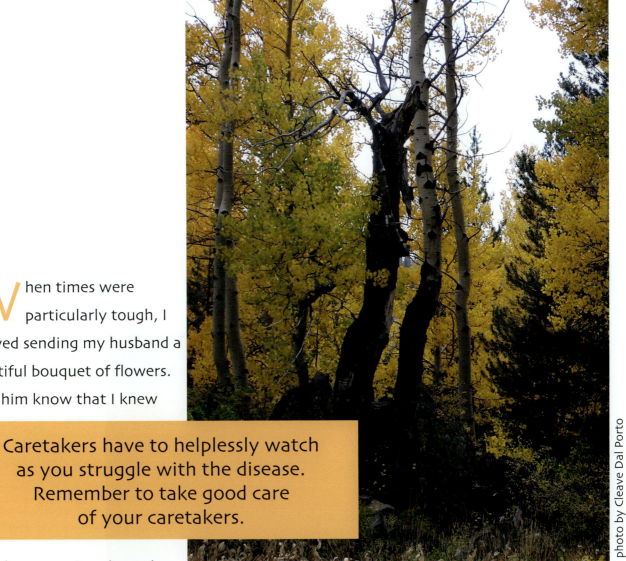

photo by Cleave Dal Porto

When times were particularly tough, I enjoyed sending my husband a beautiful bouquet of flowers. It let him know that I knew

> Caretakers have to helplessly watch as you struggle with the disease. Remember to take good care of your caretakers.

what he was going through

and it had the added bonus of a rose-scented room when he brought them home to share. And I might add ... it made the tongues wag as his fellow employees tried to figure out who was sending him flowers, and more importantly, why?

I take up to 32 pills a day. I also take naps in the warm sun, long walks with my grandchildren, laven-

**CANCER DEMANDS YOUR ATTENTION.
HOWEVER, DON'T GIVE IT YOUR HEART AND SOUL.**

der baths and time to play with my cats. And I take great pleasure in knowing that it is never too late to plan a new adventure.

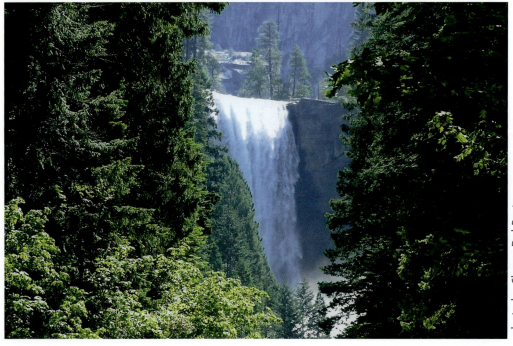

photo by Cleave Dal Porto

Shaking Hands with Cancer

After numerous surgeries behind me and without a doubt many ahead of me, I looked for ways to make these procedures more palatable. I talked with my surgeon, and found out that headsets were allowed in pre-op and

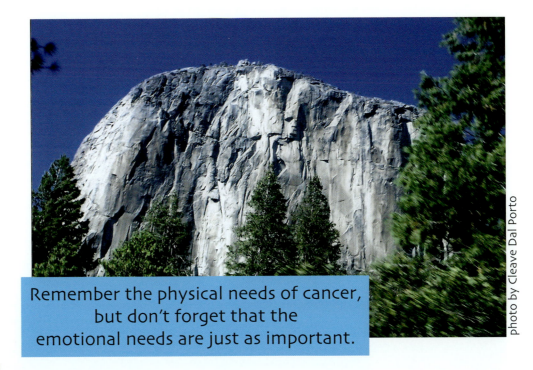

Remember the physical needs of cancer, but don't forget that the emotional needs are just as important.

although he suggested mild, soothing music, I thought my rock'-n'roll would be a way to make all of the needle poking a bit more pleasurable.

I also asked if I could bring pajamas from home and was told that as long as they were not form fitting, it would be fine. It was such a change from those drab, blue hospital gowns. My ducky pajamas also served to make patients happy. And my matching ducky slippers and robe, made people smile. I learned that you can bring your toiletries from home, and its surprising how comforting your own toothpaste and toothbrush can be. I also enjoyed my headset filled with favorite songs, my worn blanket, funny pillow cases, pictures of family, coloring books, a journal to write in and several good books. When I felt up to it, I began writing notes to some of my favorite nurses; they rarely receive the thanks they so deserve.

Even in the 21st century, it saddens me to say that prejudices are still very much in place. But er you are tall or short, young or old, heavy or thin, rich or poor, straight or gay, black, white, blue

REGARDLESS OF THE HEARTACHE,
WE MUST CHOOSE THE MOMENTS IN WHICH WE TRULY SHINE.

when it comes to prejudices, cancer has none. It can sneak into your life wheth- or purple. It is definitely an equal opportunity disease.

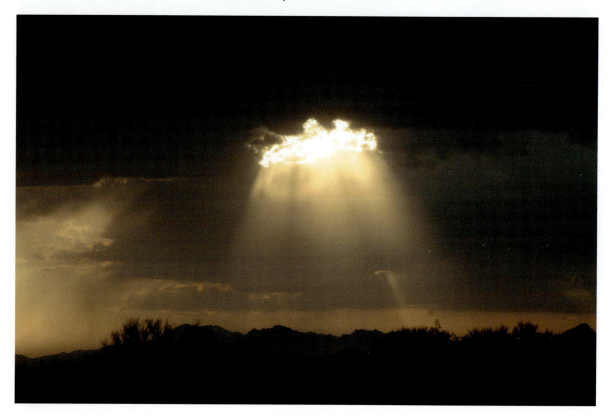

I spell my first name - cheryl - with a lower case c. The change came about ten years ago as a result of a routine appointment with my oncologist. As my doctor attended another patient, his voice heightened and I heard him say, "this is cancer with a capital C. We need to move beyond the whys and the hows, and concentrate on the what, as in what is to be our plan of action." Within moments, the doctor was standing in my examination room and he was visibly upset. He told me that "some people can't get beyond the 'this is not happening to me stage' and move forward to a plan of action." From that day forward, I began spelling my name with a lower case c. Not out of a fear of the word Cancer, with a capital C, but perhaps respect. I can still remember the doctor's words - "Cancer with a capital C." So, call it disassociating. Call it respect. Just please, spell my first name - cheryl.

Cancer taught me one of the most powerful life lessons. Horrible things happen to good people every day. It's how we handle these things that define us.

My particular cancer
took away my ability to
have intercourse. How-
ever, my husband and I
remember, with fondness,

WHEN LIFE GIVES YOU LEMONS, MAKE LEMONADE AND SHARE THE PITCHER WITH THE WORLD.

the days when we were
sexually active. Now, in
bed, we hold each other
more tightly than ever
before.

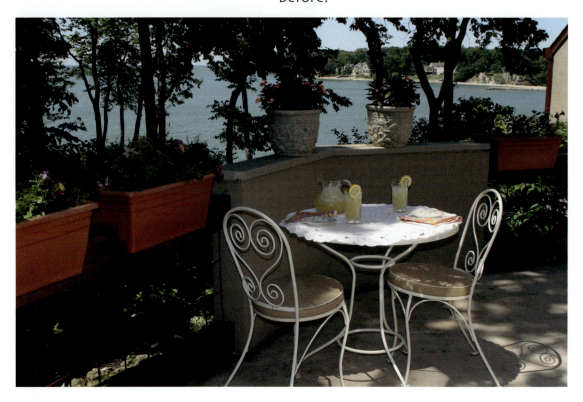

Just the other day, I saw a woman shopping. I noticed her immediately, because she was dressed in striking hues of orange. I just couldn't take my eyes off her! It was apparent that she was either in the midst of chemotherapy or had recently completed it because of the scarf wrapped neatly over her hairless head. I had to meet her. She told me she had just completed her six-week chemotherapy and lost all of her long, red hair. I told her my story. Together, just for a brief moment, we hugged. Then she thanked me for asking about her. She said that no one asked, even though her headdress made it almost impossible not to know she was fighting the battle of her life. I left the store knowing that she was going to beat her cancer and a unique person would live on to bring beauty to the world.

My grandsons tell me that they have one normal grandma and one crazy one. I am so glad that they see me as the latter.

Immediately upon waking from my latest surgery, less than a year ago, my oncology/surgeon

When I think of all the wonderful people I have met in both the oncology and radiology

I AM FILLED WITH HOPE FOR FUTURE GENERATION CANCER PATIENTS AND AM CONFIDENT THAT A CURE FOR ALL CANCERS IS ON THE HORIZON.

was holding my hand, and telling anyone who would listen to him, about the years we have been together as a doctor/patient team.

departments, I shudder to think what my life would have been without them. They are not just casual acquaintances; they are family.

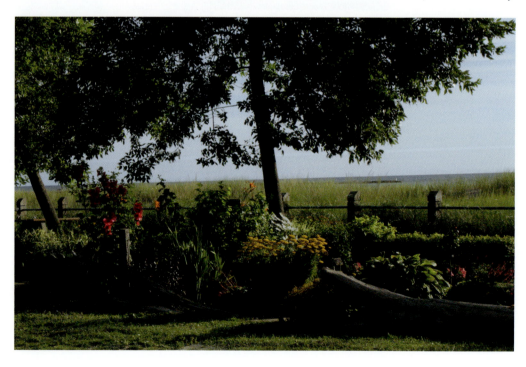

Shaking Hands with Cancer

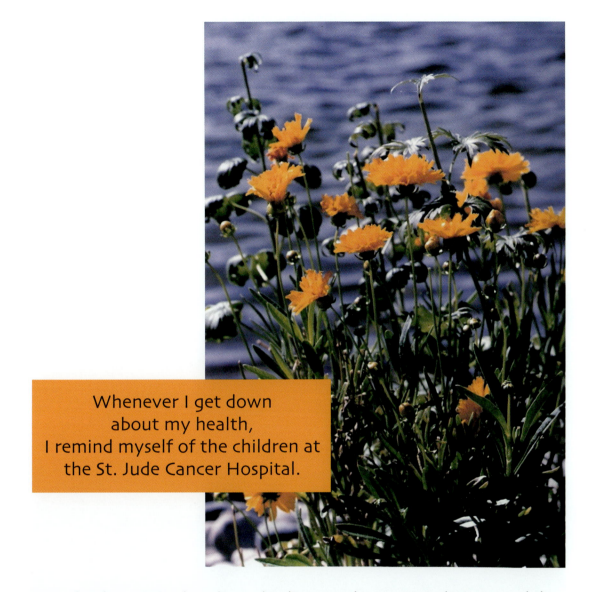

Whenever I get down
about my health,
I remind myself of the children at
the St. Jude Cancer Hospital.

Life allows you to be the writer, the editor, the director, the costume designer and the choreographer - you have a big hand in writing your own story. Make "your story" one of inspiration for others to follow. Allow the cancer one chapter in your book .... but only one chapter.

One day I didn't have cancer ... the next day I did. Now I think of events in my life as pre-cancer life. Flowers smell sweeter, children laugh louder, food tastes better and rainy days cause you to

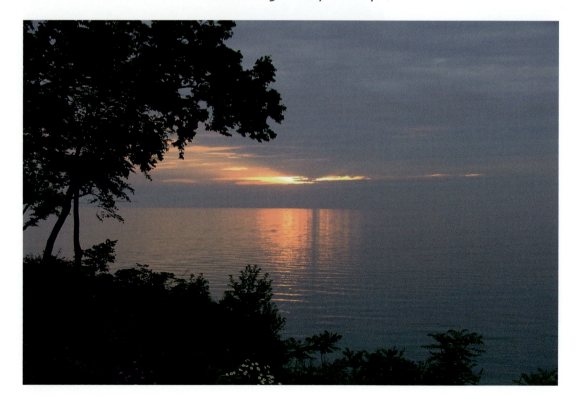

BELIEVE THAT ANYTHING IS POSSIBLE.

and post-cancer. My post-cancer days have been some of the most meaningful days of my run outside to drink in the moisture. Why? You have faced cancer and beaten it for one more day.

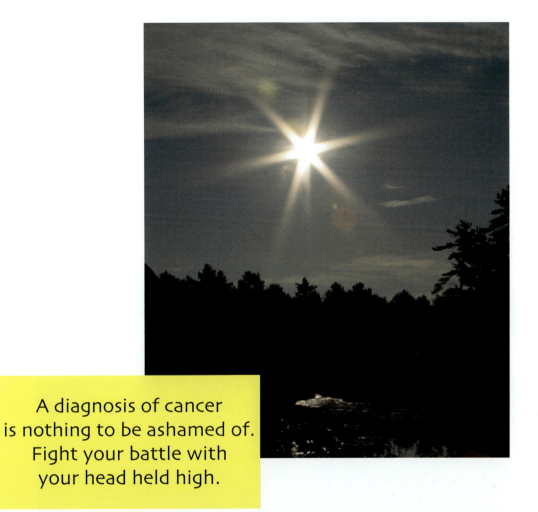

A diagnosis of cancer
is nothing to be ashamed of.
Fight your battle with
your head held high.

Even though I received a death sentence with my diagnosis of cancer (mesothelioma - a slow growing, terminal cancer), I quickly came to realize that there are worse ways to die. I am surrounded by a miraculous medical team who will do just about anything for me and I have learned to thank the universe for each new day, surrounded by friends and family, by plants and flowers, by devoted pets, by spring showers and warm, sunny days.

I once read that it is a
documented phenomenon
in modern medical practice
that people who accept a

**DON'T ALLOW THIS UNCONTROLLED GROWTH
TO CONTROL YOUR LIFE.**

cancer diagnosis as a death
sentence can die quite
quickly, long before the
disease has progressed far
enough to cause death it-
self. You can literally scare
yourself to death.

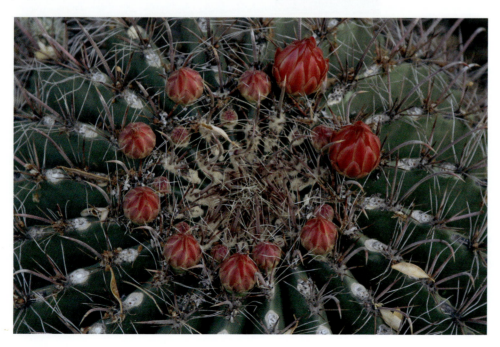

Shaking Hands with Cancer

When I was only 25 years old, my Father - one of the most important people in my life - died suddenly of a massive, heart attack. At the age of 57, he retired in June, and by November, 9 short days after his birthday, he was dead. At the time, by-passes were

Cancer can cut your life short.
So can automobile accidents, fatal heart attacks, drowning, homicide, earthquakes, childhood diseases, starvation.
With cancer, you usually get a chance to fight.

rarely done, and my Dad was told to go home ... he might live for a day, he might live for many years, no one could say. One day, he was on the 9th hole of a favorite golf course, just starting to enjoy his retirement years, and the next, he was dead. He was not given the opportunity to fight for his life. There was nothing that he or my Mother could do; my Dad was, quite literally, handed a death sentence.

I have always been thankful for the opportunity - yes, the gift - of a good fight.

I became less of a vic-
tim and took back control
of my life the day I shook
hands with my cancers,

LOOK CAREFULLY AT THE WORD CANCER
AND REALIZE THAT THE FIRST 3 LETTERS SPELL OUT - CAN.

and announced to the
world that I accepted my
opponent and vowed to
beat "it" ... perhaps not in
every round, but certainly
in the war.

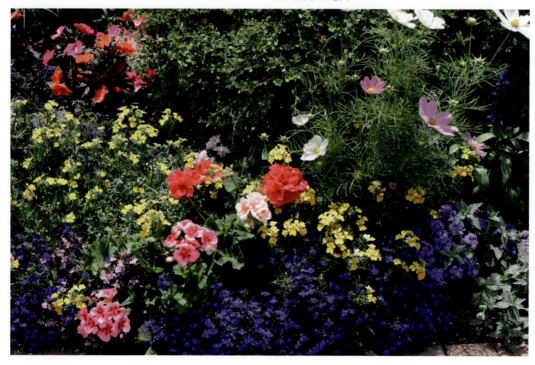

Shaking Hands with Cancer

I have heard many a cancer patient say that they are anxious to get their treatments behind them, and then return to their lives. Cancer doesn't stop your life; it's part of it.

During treatments, stay connected with those things that make your life unique. Don't put on hold the things you love. You may

A diagnosis of cancer
does not need to be the end of your path.
It can lead to a new beginning.
Your path awaits you.
What direction will you take?

not be able to perform physical activities as you did before the cancer, but you can take that first step immediately and the next day it will be two.

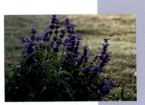 OTHER SOURCES OF HELP

Change Your Life Without Getting Out of Bed. By SARK.

Chicken Soup for the Soul: The Cancer Book: 101 Stories of Courage, Support & Love. By Jack Canfield, Mark Victor Hansen, David Tabatsky.

Crazy Sexy Cancer Survivor: More Rebellion and Fire for Your Healing Journey. By Kris Carr.

Everyone's Guide to Cancer Therapy: How Cancer is Diagnosed, Treated, and Managed: Day to Day, Revised 5th Editon. By Andrew Ko, M.D., Malin Dollinger M.D., Ernest H. Rosenbaum, M.D.

Everyone's Guide to Cancer Survivorship: A Road Map for Better Health. By R.N. Holly Gautier, David Spiegel, M.D., Ernest H. Rosenbaum, M.D.

Inner Fire: Your Will to Live. By Ernest H. Rosenbaum, M.D. and Isadora R. Rosenbaum.

The Gift of the Magi. By O. Henry.

The Great Classics - your choice. All of those wonderful books and movies you were always going to read and watch.

The Little Engine That Could. By Watty Piper. Illustrated by George Hauman and Doris Hauman.

Photography Books - your choice.

Poetry Books - your choice.

Travel Books - once you are diagnosed, immediately plan a trip for one year in the future. Then read about your destination, and dream, dream, dream!

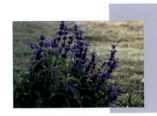

ABOUT THE AUTHOR

cheryl Dal Porto was born in Modesto, California and remained in this central California town until leaving for college in San Francisco. This was the infamous 60's and she met her first husband on the corner of Haight-Ashbury. She and her first husband had two children, Cleave, now married with two children of his own, and Marc, also married. After re-locating to Sacramento, California for a job, cheryl's first husband died. While working at the Sacramento County Sheriff's Department, she met her second husband, Bob, and together they blended their families. Now they enjoy five grandchildren and one great-grandson.

cheryl has run a successful family-owned publishing company, has led a commercial llama pack string in the Pt. Reyes National Seashore, and is currently working on The Cancer Workbook. She lives in Placerville, California, with her husband and a variety of farm animals.

ABOUT THE PHOTOGRAPHERS

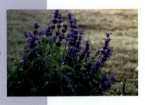

A professional photographer for over 33 years, Susan Ley specializes in animals and scenics. She is currently working on a book for amateur pet photographers titled, Digital Pet Photography. She lives in Key Largo, Florida where she enjoys the turquoise waters with her husband, Jack, and their Irish Terrier, Morgan. Please visit her web site, www.susanleyphotography to enjoy some wonderful photographs and learn tips for making your own images even better.

Cleave Dal Porto, cheryl's son, lives with his wife and two sons in Jackson, California. An amateur photographer, he enjoys taking photographs while hiking the numerous trails in Northern California.